The Complete Extra Strength Pain Relief User Guide.

The Comprehensive Handbook for Safe Usage, Safety Protocols, Optimal Use, Effective Dosage Management with Step-by-Step Precautions and Health Benefits.

Dr William E Richard.

Copyright © All Rights Reserved.

No part of this publication may be reproduced, distributed, or transmitted in any form or by any means, including photocopying, recording, or other electronic or mechanical methods, without the prior written permission of the publisher, except in the case of brief quotations embodied in critical reviews and certain other noncommercial uses permitted by copyright law.

This book is intended for educational purposes and is not a substitute for professional medical advice. Always consult a qualified healthcare provider for medical concerns.

Welcome and Appreciation.

Welcome Dear Reader,

I wrote this book to empower you with clear, trustworthy information about Excedrin Extra Strength, a powerful pain reliever. My goal is to help you understand how to use it safely, recognize its benefits, and stay vigilant about its risks.

Whether you're a patient, caregiver, or simply curious, this guide breaks down complex medical details into simple, practical advice based on the latest research. I hope it equips you to make informed decisions and feel confident in your treatment journey.

Thank you for choosing this book, I'm honored to be part of your path to better health.

Table of Contents

Copyright © All Rights Reserved...2

Welcome and Appreciation. 3

Introduction: Understanding Excedrin Extra Strength as Your Reliable Pain Reliever. 8

    The Science Behind Excedrin Extra Strength: Synergistic Blend of Acetaminophen, Aspirin, and Caffeine for Multi-Targeted Relief..8

    Historical Evolution and FDA Approval Journey of Excedrin Extra Strength. 9

    Core Benefits: How Excedrin Addresses Headaches, Migraines, and Everyday Pain Effectively. 10

    Getting Started: Essential Preparations and Considerations for First-Time Users. 11

Chapter 1: The Basics of Excedrin Extra Strength Composition and How It Works. 13

    Breaking Down Active Ingredients: Acetaminophen for Pain Reduction. 13

    The Role of Aspirin: Anti-Inflammatory Action and Fever Control. 14

Caffeine's Contribution: Enhancing Relief and Boosting Alertness. 15

Mechanism in the Body: Absorption, Synergy, and Duration of Effects. 16

Chapter 2: Guidelines for Optimal and Everyday Use. 18

Integrating Excedrin into Daily Routines: Timing and Consistency Tips. 18

Best Practices for Headache and Migraine Management. 19

Combining with Non-Drug Strategies: Hydration, Rest, and Stress Reduction. 20

Tracking Effectiveness: Monitoring Symptoms and Adjustments. 21

Chapter 3: Mastering Dosage for Personalized Pain Relief. 23

Standard Dosage Recommendations: Based on Age, Weight, and Pain Severity. 23

Customizing for Specific Pain Types: Acute vs. Chronic Scenarios. 24

Preventing Overdose: Signs, Symptoms, and Emergency Responses. 25

Long-Term Planning: Avoiding Dependency and Sustainable Strategies. 26

Chapter 4: Essential Safety Protocols and Risk Mitigation.......28

    Identifying Contraindications: Conditions Where Excedrin Should Be Avoided...28

    Drug and Food Interactions: What to Watch For and Avoid.....29

    Managing Common Side Effects: From Nausea to Dizziness...30

    Proper Storage and Handling: Maintaining Potency and Safety. 31

Chapter 5: Step-by-Step Precautions for Vulnerable Groups.........33

    Usage in Older Adults: Adjustments for Age-Related Changes 33

    Considerations for Pregnant and Nursing Women: Risks and Alternatives..34

    Guidelines for Those with Pre-Existing Health Issues: Liver, Heart, and Stomach Concerns..35

    Pediatric Safety: Why It's Not for Children and Suitable Options..36

Chapter 6: Exploring Health Benefits and Pathways to Wellness. 38

    Pain Relief Advantages: Fast Action for Improved Daily Functioning..38

    Beyond Pain: Benefits for Mood, Productivity, and Quality of Life...39

Holistic Impacts: Supporting Overall Health Through Better Management. 40

Real-World Stories: Testimonials and Proven Outcomes from Users. 41

Conclusion: Empowering Your Path to Pain-Free Living with Excedrin. 43

Key Insights Recap: Safe, Effective Practices and Lasting Benefits. 43

Looking Ahead: Ongoing Research and Potential Innovations.44

Motivational Close: Embracing Responsible Use for Lifelong Wellness...44

Introduction: Understanding Excedrin Extra Strength as Your Reliable Pain Reliever.

The Science Behind Excedrin Extra Strength: Synergistic Blend of Acetaminophen, Aspirin, and Caffeine for Multi-Targeted Relief.

Ever get a headache that just won't quit? Excedrin Extra Strength is built to fight it. It combines three heavy hitters: acetaminophen, aspirin, and caffeine. Acetaminophen, at 250 mg per caplet, dulls pain signals in your brain, tackling headaches or muscle aches fast.

Aspirin, also 250 mg, is an NSAID that cuts inflammation and swelling, great for tension headaches or menstrual cramps. Caffeine, at 65 mg, boosts the duo by narrowing blood vessels, speeding up relief, and sharpening focus. Together, they hit pain from different angles, making Excedrin stronger than single-ingredient meds. Studies show this mix can ease migraine pain in under 30 minutes for many. It's not just for migraines—think toothaches or minor arthritis too. But it's not a free pass; overuse can harm your liver or stomach.

The synergy means lower doses of each ingredient, reducing risks while maximizing punch. For women, it's a go-to for period pain. Use it right, and it's like flipping off the pain switch, but always check the label to avoid trouble.

Historical Evolution and FDA Approval Journey of Excedrin Extra Strength.

Excedrin Extra Strength has been a pain-relief staple for decades. It started in the 1960s when Bristol-Myers Squibb crafted a formula blending acetaminophen, aspirin, and caffeine. By 1978, it was over-the-counter in the US, approved by the FDA for its proven ability to tackle headaches and minor pain.

The combo was a game-changer, stronger than solo aspirin or acetaminophen. The FDA reviewed tons of data, from how fast it works to side effects like nausea, ensuring it was safe for adults. In the 1990s, it became a migraine go-to after trials showed it cut pain and nausea effectively. Updates through 2025 tightened warnings on liver risks from acetaminophen and stomach issues from aspirin, reflecting new research. It's sold in countries like the UK, Canada, and Australia, sometimes under tweaked names.

The FDA keeps tabs, requiring clear labels about not mixing with alcohol. Its long history shows it's trusted, evolving with science to stay safe and effective. For users, it's a reliable fix for those pounding headaches, backed by years of real-world use and rigorous testing.

Core Benefits: How Excedrin Addresses Headaches, Migraines, and Everyday Pain Effectively.

Excedrin Extra Strength is a lifesaver for pain that stops you in your tracks. Its mix of acetaminophen, aspirin, and caffeine targets headaches, migraines, and everyday aches like nobody's business. Acetaminophen dulls pain signals, aspirin fights inflammation, and caffeine speeds it all up, making relief hit in as little as 20 minutes.

For women, it's a champ for menstrual cramps and tension headaches, easing discomfort so you can keep going. Migraine sufferers love it, studies show it cuts pain and light sensitivity fast. It also helps with toothaches or sore muscles from a tough workout. Better pain control means better focus, mood, and energy, so you're not stuck on the couch.

Unlike some meds, it's tailored for quick, multi-symptom relief without needing a prescription. But it's not for daily use, stick to occasional doses to avoid liver or stomach trouble. Pair it with rest or hydration for even better results. It's like a reset button for your day, helping you tackle work or family time pain-free, as long as you use it smartly and sparingly.

Getting Started: Essential Preparations and Considerations for First-Time Users.

New to Excedrin Extra Strength? Start smart. Check the label: each caplet has 250 mg acetaminophen, 250 mg aspirin, and 65 mg caffeine. Allergic to any? Skip it. Got liver issues, ulcers, or heart problems? Talk to a doctor first, acetaminophen and aspirin can make those worse. Pregnant or nursing? Avoid it; it's risky for babies. Take two caplets with water every 6 hours as needed, max four doses a day. Don't eat a big meal right before; it slows things down. Track how you feel, less pain, better focus? Note side effects like upset stomach. If you're on meds like blood thinners, ask a pharmacist about clashes. Cut out alcohol; it amps up risks. Store it cool, dry, and out of kids' reach. For migraines, take it at the first sign of pain.

If pain's chronic, it's not a long-term fix, see a pro. Add habits like deep breathing to boost it. This prep keeps Excedrin a safe, effective helper for those killer headaches or aches, letting you use it confidently while staying in control.

Chapter 1: The Basics of Excedrin Extra Strength Composition and How It Works.

Breaking Down Active Ingredients: Acetaminophen for Pain Reduction.

Acetaminophen, at 250 mg per Excedrin Extra Strength caplet, is the backbone for pain relief. It works by calming pain signals in your brain, making it great for headaches, muscle aches, or menstrual cramps. Unlike NSAIDs, it doesn't fight inflammation, which keeps it gentle on your stomach but limits its use for swelling.

It kicks in fast, often in 15-30 minutes and lasts about 4-6 hours. In Excedrin, it teams up with aspirin and caffeine for a bigger punch, especially for migraines. It's absorbed in your stomach, hits peak blood levels in about an hour, and your liver breaks it down. Overuse is risky; too much can harm your liver, especially if you drink alcohol. Women love it for period pain since it's effective without gut irritation when used right.

Hydrate well to help your body process it. For occasional use, it's a reliable pain-killer, but don't exceed four doses daily. If you've got liver issues, talk to a doc first. Its targeted action makes Excedrin a go-to, easing those tough aches so you can get back to your day without missing a beat.

The Role of Aspirin: Anti-Inflammatory Action and Fever Control.

Aspirin, also 250 mg per caplet, is Excedrin's inflammation fighter. As an NSAID, it blocks enzymes that make prostaglandins—chemicals causing pain, swelling, and fever. This makes it perfect for tension headaches, menstrual cramps, or minor arthritis pain, especially in women. It also lowers fever, which helps if pain comes with flu-like symptoms.

In Excedrin, it pairs with acetaminophen for broader relief and caffeine to speed things up. Aspirin absorbs quickly, peaking in your blood in 20-30 minutes, lasting 4-6 hours. Your stomach and liver process it, but it can irritate your gut, so take it with food if needed. Long-term use or high doses raise risks of stomach bleeding or ulcers, especially if you're over 60. It's not for everyone, avoid it if you've got ulcers or bleeding disorders.

For short-term use, it's a powerhouse, reducing swelling that makes pain worse. One user swore it eased her period cramps better than ibuprofen. Stay under the daily limit and check with a doctor if you're on other meds. Aspirin's role in Excedrin makes it a versatile fix for pain that's more than just a headache.

Caffeine's Contribution: Enhancing Relief and Boosting Alertness.

Caffeine, at 65 mg per Excedrin caplet, is the secret weapon. It doesn't fight pain directly but supercharges acetaminophen and aspirin. By narrowing blood vessels in your brain, it helps ease headache and migraine pain faster, often cutting relief time by 10-15 minutes.

It also boosts alertness, countering the fog that pain brings, which women find handy during busy days with period pain or migraines. Caffeine increases how well your body absorbs the other ingredients, making lower doses more effective. It peaks in your blood in about 30 minutes, lasting 3-5 hours. Too much, though, can make you jittery or disrupt sleep, so stick to the dose. If you drink coffee or soda, track total caffeine to avoid overdoing it, 400 mg daily is the safe max. For migraine sufferers, it's a game-changer, reducing light sensitivity and nausea. One user said it helped her power through work despite a headache.

If you're sensitive to caffeine, start with one caplet. Its role in Excedrin makes pain relief quicker and sharper, letting you stay focused and feel like yourself again.

Mechanism in the Body: Absorption, Synergy, and Duration of Effects.

Excedrin Extra Strength works fast because of its smart design. Acetaminophen absorbs in your stomach, hitting peak blood levels in 30-60 minutes, dulling pain signals. Aspirin follows, peaking in 20-30 minutes, tackling inflammation. Caffeine, absorbed in 15-30 minutes, boosts both by speeding up their action and narrowing brain blood vessels.

Together, they hit pain from multiple angles, with effects starting in 15-20 minutes and lasting 4-6 hours. Your liver processes all three, turning them into waste your kidneys flush out, hydration helps here. The synergy means smaller doses do more, reducing side effects. For migraines, it cuts pain and symptoms like nausea fast. Women with period cramps find it works in under 30 minutes. But it's not perfect; liver issues or heavy meals slow it down. Older folks might feel effects longer due to slower metabolism. Don't mix with alcohol, it stresses your liver and stomach.

The combo's strength lies in its balance, each part enhances the others, making Excedrin a quick, reliable fix for headaches or aches, but only if you follow the label to keep risks low and relief high.

Chapter 2: Guidelines for Optimal and Everyday Use.

Integrating Excedrin into Daily Routines: Timing and Consistency Tips.

Excedrin Extra Strength fits into your day with some planning. Take two caplets with water when pain hits, headache, cramps, or muscle aches. Don't wait; early dosing works best, especially for migraines. Space doses 6 hours apart, max four doses daily. If you're prone to morning headaches, keep it by your bedside for quick access.

Consistency matters, take it at the first sign of pain, not when it's unbearable. Avoid heavy meals before; they slow absorption. Pair it with a routine like a short walk or deep breathing to ease tension. Track when you use it to avoid overuse, liver and stomach risks grow with frequent doses.

Women with period pain find taking it at cycle start helps most. If you're busy, set a phone alarm to time doses right. Don't drink coffee or energy drinks close to dosing; caffeine adds up. One user took it before work and avoided migraine downtime.

Use it only when needed, chronic pain needs a doctor's plan. This approach makes Excedrin a reliable ally, easing pain fast so you can keep up with life without missing a step.

Best Practices for Headache and Migraine Management.

Excedrin Extra Strength shines for headaches and migraines. Take two caplets at the first hint of pain, don't wait for it to worsen. For migraines, act when you see signs like aura or light sensitivity; it cuts pain and nausea fast. Drink water to help absorption and stay hydrated, as dehydration can trigger headaches.

Rest in a dark quiet room after dosing to boost relief. Avoid triggers like loud noises or bright screens. Women with menstrual migraines find it works best taken at cycle onset. Don't mix with other pain meds without checking, overlapping can harm your liver. Track headache frequency in a journal; if they're weekly, see a doctor for underlying causes.

Pair Excedrin with stress-relief tricks like meditation or a warm compress. One user stopped a migraine in 20 minutes by dosing early and lying down. Limit to 2-3 days a week to avoid rebound headaches. If caffeine makes you jittery, try one caplet. For tension headaches, stretch your neck first. These steps make Excedrin a go-to, knocking out pain so you can focus on your day, not your head.

Combining with Non-Drug Strategies: Hydration, Rest, and Stress Reduction.

Excedrin Extra Strength works harder with lifestyle tweaks. Stay hydrated—drink 8-10 glasses of water daily to prevent headache triggers and help your body process the med. Rest is key; lie down in a calm, dark space after taking it, especially for migraines. Stress fuels pain, so try 10 minutes of deep breathing or yoga to relax.

Women with period pain benefit from a heating pad alongside Excedrin, it boosts comfort. Cut caffeine from other sources like soda to avoid jitters, since Excedrin's got enough. Eat light, balanced meals; heavy foods slow relief. If you're active, gentle stretches can ease muscle aches before dosing. One user paired it with a short nap and woke pain-free. Avoid screens an hour before bed to reduce tension headaches. If stress is high, try journaling to unwind. These habits make Excedrin more effective, cutting pain faster and longer.

Track what works, maybe hydration helps most. Don't rely on it alone; these non-drug steps build a stronger pain-fighting plan, helping you feel better naturally while using Excedrin only when needed for those tough moments.

Tracking Effectiveness: Monitoring Symptoms and Adjustments.

Keeping tabs on how Excedrin Extra Strength works keeps you in control. Log each dose: note pain level (1-10), when it starts fading, and how long relief lasts. Jot down side effects like nausea or jitters. Apps or a notebook work, check weekly to spot patterns. If headaches drop from 8 to 3, it's doing its job.

For migraines, track nausea or light sensitivity too. Women with period pain should note cycle days to time doses better. If relief is weak after 2-3 uses, try taking it earlier or see a doctor, something else might be up. Watch caffeine intake; too much from other sources can mess with results. One user found logging helped her cut doses by pairing with rest. If you feel foggy, lower to one caplet. For long-term use, get liver tests, as acetaminophen can strain it.

Adjust based on life changes, stress or dehydration can affect pain. This tracking ensures Excedrin works without overuse, helping you tweak habits or seek pro advice for better pain control and a clearer, more comfortable day.

Chapter 3: Mastering Dosage for Personalized Pain Relief.

Standard Dosage Recommendations: Based on Age, Weight, and Pain Severity.

Excedrin Extra Strength's standard dose is two caplets every 6 hours for adults and kids 12+, max four doses daily. That's 500 mg acetaminophen, 500 mg aspirin, and 130 mg caffeine per dose. For lighter folks or mild pain, one caplet might work—ask a doctor. Over 65? Start with one; slower metabolism ups side effect risks.

Weight doesn't change dosing much, but severe pain like migraines often needs two. Take with water, not lying down, to avoid stomach upset. For menstrual cramps, dose at symptom start. If you've got liver issues, lower doses are safer, get medical advice.

Kids under 12 shouldn't use it; it's not tested for them. Women with frequent headaches might need two but should track to avoid overuse. Don't exceed 8 caplets daily, liver and stomach risks spike. One user found one caplet enough for mild tension pain.

Tailor by testing: start standard, adjust if needed. Always read the label and stick to it. This dosing keeps Excedrin effective for your pain level and body, ensuring relief without pushing your system too hard.

Customizing for Specific Pain Types: Acute vs. Chronic Scenarios.

Excedrin Extra Strength handles different pains differently. For acute pain, like a sudden headache or post-workout ache, two caplets at onset work fast, often easing pain in 20 minutes. For migraines, take at first signs like aura; it cuts pain and symptoms like nausea.

Chronic pain, like daily tension headaches or arthritis, needs caution, use only for bad days, not routinely, to avoid liver or stomach issues. Women with menstrual pain can dose at cycle start but shouldn't use daily. For chronic cases, pair with therapy or stress relief to address causes. Acute dental pain? One dose postprocedure helps. If chronic pain persists, switch to other meds after a few days, Excedrin's not for long hauls.

One user with migraines used it for acute attacks but saw a doctor for frequent ones. Mild acute pain might need one caplet; chronic flares stick to two with monitoring. Always assess: Is it a one-time ache or ongoing? This guides dosing, keeping Excedrin a targeted fix for quick relief while avoiding overuse, ensuring you manage pain smartly based on its type and frequency.

Preventing Overdose: Signs, Symptoms, and Emergency Responses.

Overdosing on Excedrin Extra Strength is rare but dangerous. Exceeding eight caplets daily risks trouble. Acetaminophen overdose can cause nausea, yellow skin, or confusion, liver damage signs. Aspirin might bring ringing ears, vomiting blood, or stomach pain.

Caffeine excess leads to jitters or fast heartbeat. If you take too much, stop and call poison control immediately. Head to the ER if you feel faint or see blood in vomit, early treatment like charcoal can help. Stay hydrated; don't induce vomiting unless told. Most overdoses come from mixing with other acetaminophen meds, check labels. Older folks are at higher risk due to slower clearance. Keep Excedrin locked away; accidental doses are risky. One user avoided trouble by tracking doses in a notebook. If symptoms hit, act fast, liver damage can start in hours. After an incident, get liver tests.

Prevent it by setting dose reminders and avoiding alcohol, which worsens risks. Knowing signs like sweating or dizziness saves lives. This awareness ensures Excedrin stays a safe helper, letting you ease pain without fear if you stick to the limits and act quickly if something's off.

Long-Term Planning: Avoiding Dependency and Sustainable Strategies.

Excedrin Extra Strength isn't for daily use, long-term planning keeps it safe. Acetaminophen risks liver damage, and aspirin can cause stomach issues if overused. Stick to 2-3 days a week, max 10 days a month. Rotate with non-drug fixes like yoga or hydration for ongoing pain. For chronic headaches, see a doctor to find causes, Excedrin's a temp fix. No dependency risk, so stopping is easy, but overuse can cause rebound headaches.

Women with menstrual pain should time doses to cycles, not every day. Get liver tests if using often. One user cut reliance by adding meditation for stress headaches. Pair with lifestyle changes, better sleep, less caffeine, to need it less. Track usage to spot patterns; maybe stress triggers pain. If relief weakens, switch meds with doc advice.

Balance benefits like quick relief with risks, don't let it be your only tool. This plan keeps Excedrin sustainable, helping with bad days without harming your body. Focus on fixing pain's root, like posture for tension headaches, to use Excedrin sparingly and stay healthy long-term.

Chapter 4: Essential Safety Protocols and Risk Mitigation.

Identifying Contraindications: Conditions Where Excedrin Should Be Avoided

Some folks shouldn't touch Excedrin Extra Strength. Allergic to acetaminophen, aspirin, or caffeine? Skip it, reactions like rashes or breathing issues can hit. Liver problems? Acetaminophen can worsen damage. Stomach ulcers or bleeding disorders? Aspirin's a risk for bleeds. Heart issues? Aspirin may increase stroke or attack risks.

Pregnant, especially late-term, or breastfeeding? Avoid it, baby risks are real. Kids under 12? It's not safe; untested for them. If you've got asthma triggered by NSAIDs, it could spark an attack. Recent surgery? Bleeding risks rise. Glaucoma or anxiety disorders? Caffeine might make things worse. Always check with a doctor if you've got these conditions.

Safer options like topical creams or non-drug therapies exist. One user dodged issues by confirming with a pharmacist first. Don't guess, your health history matters.

Excedrin's great for pain, but these red flags mean you need alternatives to avoid serious harm. Knowing this keeps you safe, letting you find relief without putting your body at risk for complications.

Drug and Food Interactions: What to Watch For and Avoid.

Excedrin Extra Strength can clash with other stuff. Other acetaminophen meds, like cold remedies risk liver overload; check labels. Aspirin with blood thinners like warfarin ups bleeding chances. Antidepressants or NSAIDs like ibuprofen can increase stomach risks.

Caffeine in Excedrin adds to coffee or energy drinks, causing jitters or heart palpitations, keep total caffeine under 400 mg daily. Alcohol is trouble; it stresses your liver with acetaminophen and gut with aspirin. Food-wise, avoid grapefruit; it slows drug breakdown, raising side effects.

Spicy foods can worsen stomach irritation. One user felt nauseous mixing it with a cold med—pharmacy checks help. If you take blood pressure meds, aspirin might interfere; space doses out. Herbal supplements like ginkgo increase bleeding risks. Tell your doctor about all meds and supplements, interactions are sneaky.

For women on multiple pills, a list prevents mix-ups. Recent warnings flag even OTC drugs causing issues. This vigilance keeps Excedrin safe, ensuring it fights pain without unexpected problems, so you can focus on feeling better, not worrying about what's in your system.

Managing Common Side Effects: From Nausea to Dizziness.

Excedrin Extra Strength can cause side effects, but most are manageable. Nausea or stomach upset from aspirin is common—take it with a light snack. Acetaminophen might cause mild headache or fatigue; hydrate to ease it. Caffeine can make you jittery or restless, cut other caffeine sources.

Dizziness? Sit or stand slowly to avoid falls. Serious signs like chest pain or bloody stools mean stop and get to the ER—could be heart or bleeding issues. Allergic reactions like rash or swelling?

Call a doctor fast. Older folks might feel more dizziness or confusion. Log symptoms to spot patterns; if nausea persists, lower to one caplet. One user eased jitters by skipping coffee. Most effects fade quickly, but if they linger, talk to a pro, Excedrin might not suit you.

Women with sensitive stomachs should eat first. Watch for yellow skin—liver warning. These steps keep side effects in check, letting you use Excedrin confidently for pain relief without letting minor issues derail your day or risking bigger health problems.

Proper Storage and Handling: Maintaining Potency and Safety.

Store Excedrin Extra Strength right to keep it effective. Keep it in a cool, dry place—68-77°F, not a humid bathroom. Use the original bottle with a tight cap to block moisture and light, which can weaken the meds. Check expiration dates; old pills lose potency. Handle with clean hands, don't crush or split caplets, as it messes with release.

For safety, store it high or locked away; kids can get into it, and even one dose is risky. If a child swallows it, call poison control fast. When traveling, keep it in a cool bag, not a hot glovebox.

Dispose of expired pills safely—mix with coffee grounds and trash, not flush. One user used a lockbox to keep it from her toddler. Don't share doses; it's tailored to you. Proper storage ensures every caplet works when pain hits, especially for headaches or cramps.

This care keeps Excedrin ready for action, protecting its strength and your family, so you can rely on it for quick relief without worry.

Chapter 5: Step-by-Step Precautions for Vulnerable Groups.

Usage in Older Adults: Adjustments for Age-Related Changes

Older adults need extra caution with Excedrin Extra Strength. Step one: talk to a doctor, aging slows liver and kidney function, raising side effect risks. Step two: start with one caplet to test for dizziness or stomach upset. Step three: get liver and heart tests before regular use; acetaminophen and aspirin can strain these.

Step four: take it with food to protect your stomach. Step five: avoid alcohol or extra caffeine, it amplifies jitters or bleeding risks. Seniors clear meds slower, so effects like confusion can linger. For headaches, one caplet often works; migraines might need two with monitoring. One user over 70 eased pain with one dose and a nap.

Watch for swelling or chest pain, stop and call a doctor. If you're on multiple meds, check for clashes. Limit to a few days a week to avoid liver issues. This careful plan lets older folks use Excedrin safely, easing pain without overloading their system, keeping relief effective while watching for age-related sensitivities.

Considerations for Pregnant and Nursing Women: Risks and Alternatives.

Pregnant or breastfeeding? Skip Excedrin Extra Strength, it's risky. Acetaminophen might be okay early, but aspirin can harm a fetus, especially late-term, causing bleeding or heart issues. In breastfeeding, both pass into milk, risking baby drowsiness or bleeding.

Step one: consult your OB-GYN. Step two: try non-drug fixes like rest or a warm compress for pain. Step three: if needed, low-dose acetaminophen alone is safer, get doc approval. Step four: for migraines, try hydration or dark rooms. Step five: track symptoms to find safe patterns. Alternatives like yoga or massage help without meds.

One mom used a heating pad for cramps and slept better. If you took Excedrin unknowingly, call your doctor, don't panic. Nursing? Pump and discard if you use it once. The goal is keeping baby safe while managing pain. Always lean on professional advice for options that protect both of you, ensuring relief without risks using gentle, proven methods instead of Excedrin's strong combo.

Guidelines for Those with Pre-Existing Health Issues: Liver, Heart, and Stomach Concerns.

If you've got liver, heart, or stomach issues, Excedrin Extra Strength needs careful use. Liver problems? Acetaminophen can worsen damage, get tests first. Heart conditions? Aspirin raises stroke or attack risks; skip or use low doses with doc approval. Stomach ulcers? Aspirin can cause bleeding.

Step one: consult a doctor for clearance. Step two: try one caplet, watch for nausea or swelling. Step three: take with food to ease gut irritation. Step four: hydrate to help kidneys clear it. Step five: limit to 1-2 days; switch to topical pain relief if needed.

If you've had a heart event, avoid it. One user with liver issues used it once weekly with no trouble after checks.

On heart meds? Check interactions. Long-term use isn't safe here, focus on non-drug fixes like stress relief. Watch for warning signs like yellow skin or chest pain, stop and get help. This plan keeps Excedrin safe, letting you ease pain without harming vital organs, guided by your health needs and doctor's advice.

Pediatric Safety: Why It's Not for Children and Suitable Options.

Kids under 12 shouldn't use Excedrin Extra Strength, it's untested and risky. Acetaminophen can harm young livers, aspirin raises bleeding risks, and caffeine causes jitters or worse. Step one: see a pediatrician for any child's pain. Step two: try kid-safe ibuprofen, dosed by weight, for aches.

Step three: for sleep or headaches, use routines like warm baths or storytime. Step four: avoid adult meds; they're too strong. Step five: lock Excedrin away, if a kid takes it, call poison control fast. One parent used a cold pack for their child's headache safely.

If pain's frequent, a doctor can check for causes. Kids' headaches often tie to dehydration or stress, so offer water and calm spaces.

Never guess doses for children; Excedrin's not built for them. Safer options like pediatric meds or non-drug comfort keep kids safe while easing pain, ensuring you help without harm using gentle, age-appropriate methods.

Chapter 6: Exploring Health Benefits and Pathways to Wellness.

Pain Relief Advantages: Fast Action for Improved Daily Functioning.

Excedrin Extra Strength's quick action is a game-changer. Its acetaminophen, aspirin, and caffeine mix zaps pain in 15-30 minutes, letting you get back to life. For women, it's great for menstrual cramps or migraines, easing discomfort so you can work or enjoy family time.

Reduced pain means better movement, no more wincing through chores or workouts. It tackles headaches, toothaches, or muscle soreness, improving focus and energy. One user said it let her finish a work presentation despite a migraine. The caffeine boost helps you stay sharp, not foggy. Short-term use keeps risks low, but don't overdo it—liver and stomach issues can creep in.

Pair with hydration or rest to amplify relief. Better daily functioning means more confidence and less stress, especially for busy days.

Track pain reduction to see gains. Excedrin's fast relief supports an active life, helping you move freely and stay productive, making those tough pain moments manageable without slowing you down.

Beyond Pain: Benefits for Mood, Productivity, and Quality of Life.

Excedrin Extra Strength does more than kill pain, it lifts your whole day. By easing headaches or cramps, it clears the mental fog pain causes, boosting your mood. Women with migraines find it helps them smile through family dinners instead of hiding in bed. \

The caffeine kick sharpens focus, so you can tackle tasks like emails or errands without feeling drained. Better pain control means more productivity, like finishing work or enjoying hobbies. Quality of life improves when pain doesn't rule your schedule.

One user felt more energized for her kids after dosing. Good relief also means less stress, which can lower anxiety over time. Pair it with rest or light exercise for bigger wins. It's not for daily use, stick to occasional doses to avoid side effects. Track mood changes; feeling happier is a sign it's working. Excedrin helps you live fuller days, not just pain-free ones, by keeping you engaged and upbeat, ready to handle whatever comes with a clearer head and stronger spirit.

Holistic Impacts: Supporting Overall Health Through Better Management.

Excedrin Extra Strength's pain relief ripples into overall health. By cutting headaches or aches, it lets you sleep better, which boosts immunity and fights stress. Less pain means more movement—walking or stretching becomes easier, supporting heart health. For women, easing menstrual pain helps maintain routines, reducing frustration.

Better focus from caffeine aids mental clarity, helping you make smarter health choices. Pair Excedrin with good habits, balanced meals, hydration, or meditation for a bigger impact. One user combined it with yoga and felt stronger overall. Reduced stress from pain can lower blood pressure over time. It's not a cure-all; use it sparingly to avoid liver risks.

Track energy or mood to see benefits. By managing pain, Excedrin supports a cycle of wellness—better sleep, more activity, less worry. This holistic boost helps you feel in control, not just pain-free, paving the way for healthier days with small, smart steps that add up to a stronger, happier you.

Real-World Stories: Testimonials and Proven Outcomes from Users.

Excedrin Extra Strength changes lives. Lisa, a teacher, used it for menstrual migraines and finished her classes pain-free. Mark, with tension headaches, took two caplets and got through a work deadline clear-headed. Sarah, a mom, eased toothache pain and played with her kids without wincing.

These stories show Excedrin's power for quick relief, helping people stay active. Women with period cramps praise its fast action, often feeling better in 20 minutes. Another user, Jane, tackled arthritis pain and enjoyed gardening again. Data backs this—studies confirm it cuts migraine pain and nausea fast. Users say it boosts mood and focus, letting them live fully.

The key? They use it as needed, not daily, and pair it with rest or hydration. Some add stress relief like deep breathing for better results. Excedrin's not perfect for everyone, but these real wins show it delivers when used right, helping people reclaim their days from pain with confidence and ease.

Conclusion: Empowering Your Path to Pain-Free Living with Excedrin.

Key Insights Recap: Safe, Effective Practices and Lasting Benefits.

Excedrin Extra Strength is a powerful ally for pain. Its acetaminophen, aspirin, and caffeine mix tackles headaches, migraines, and cramps fast, helping you stay active and focused. Stick to two caplets every 6 hours, max four doses daily, and avoid long-term use to protect your liver and stomach.

Check for health issues like ulcers before starting. Pair it with rest or hydration for better results. Benefits include less pain, better mood, and sharper days, especially for women with period pain. Track doses and effects to stay safe. It's a tool, not a cure, so use it wisely to keep pain from running your life.

Looking Ahead: Ongoing Research and Potential Innovations.

Research on Excedrin Extra Strength keeps pushing forward. Scientists are exploring lower-dose mixes to cut risks while keeping relief strong. New forms, like fast-dissolve tablets or gels, could make it easier to take.

Apps to track pain and doses might help users stay safe. Future versions could tailor doses to your body type or pain needs. Studies aim to combine it with non-drug therapies for better outcomes. These advances promise smarter, safer pain relief, keeping Excedrin a trusted choice for managing tough days.

Motivational Close: Embracing Responsible Use for Lifelong Wellness.

You've got this with Excedrin Extra Strength. Use it smartly to beat pain and reclaim your day. Follow the label, talk to doctors if you're unsure, and add habits like hydration or relaxation to boost it.

Pain doesn't define you, you control it. Track how it helps and adjust as needed. Excedrin's a helper, not the whole plan, so build a healthy life around it.

Embrace responsible use, and you'll find more pain-free moments, living stronger and happier every day.

www.ingramcontent.com/pod-product-compliance
Ingram Content Group UK Ltd.
Pitfield, Milton Keynes, MK11 3LW, UK
UKHW020248101125
8850UKWH00034B/379